Table of Contents

INTRODUCTION

Fungal nail infections are common and are caused by fungi that live in the environment. They enter through small cracks in your nail or the nearby skin, causing infection. Fungal infections can affect any part of the body. Fungi are normally present in and on the body alongside various bacteria. But when a fungus begins to overgrow, you can get an infection. Onychomycosis, also called tinea unguium, is a fungal infection that affects either the fingernails or toenails. Fungal infections normally develop over time, so any immediate difference in the way your nail looks or feels may be too subtle to notice at first.

Why does it develop?

A fungal nail infection occurs from the overgrowth of fungi in, under, or on the nail. Fungi thrive in warm, moist environments, so this type of environment can cause them to naturally overpopulate. The same fungi that cause jock itch, athlete's foot, and ringworm can cause nail infections. Fungi that are already present in or on your body can cause nail infections. If you have come in contact with someone else who has a fungal infection, you may have contracted it as well. Fungal infections affect toenails more commonly than fingernails, likely because your toes are usually confined to shoes, where they're in a warm, moist environment.

If you get a manicure or pedicure at a nail salon, be sure to ask how the staff disinfects their tools and how often they do it. Tools, such as emery boards and nail clippers, can spread fungal infections from person to person if they're not sanitized.

Who's at risk for fungal infections?

There are many different causes of fungal nail infections. Each cause has a treatment of its own. Although many of the causes of a fungal nail infection are preventable, some risk factors increase the likelihood of developing one. You're more likely to develop a fungal nail infection if you:

have diabetes

have a disease that causes poor circulation

are over age 65

wear artificial nails

swim in a public swimming pool

have a nail injury

have a skin injury around the nail

have moist fingers or toes for an extended time

have a weakened immune system

wear closed-toe shoes, such as tennis shoes or boots

Nail infections occur more often in men than in women, and the infections are found in adults more often than in children. If you have family members who often get these types of fungal infections, you're more likely to get them as well. Older adults have a high risk for getting fungal nail infections because they have poorer circulation. The nails also grow more slowly and thicken as we age.

What does it look like?

A fungal infection of the nail may affect part of the nail, the entire nail, or several nails. Common signs of a fungal nail infection include:

a distorted nail that may lift off from the nail bed

an odor coming from the infected nail

a brittle or thickened nail

What are common kinds of nail fungus?

Distal subungual infection

Distal subungual infections are the most common type of fungal nail infection and can develop in both fingernails and toenails. When infected, the outer edge of the nail has a jagged appearance with white and/or yellow streaks across the nail. The infection invades the nail bed and underside of the nail.

White superficial infection

White superficial infections usually affect toenails. A certain type of fungus attacks the top layers of the nail and creates well-defined white spots on the nail.Eventually these white patches cover the entire nail, which becomes rough, soft, and prone to crumbling. Spots on nail may become pitted and flaky.

Proximal subungual infection

Proximal subungual infections are uncommon but can affect both fingernails and toenails. Yellow spots appear at the base of the nail as the infection spreads upward. This infection can commonly occur in people with compromised immune systems. It can also result from minor injury to the nail.

Candida infection

Candida yeasts cause this type of infection. It can invade nails previously damaged by a prior infection or injury. More commonly, Candida affects fingernails. It often occurs in people who frequently soak their hands in water. These infections usually start by the cuticle around the nail, which becomes swollen, red, and tender to the touch. The nail itself may partially lift off the nail bed, or fall off completely.

How do I know if I have a fungal nail infection?

Because other infections can affect the nail and mimic symptoms of a fungal nail infection, the only way to confirm a diagnosis is to see a doctor. They'll take a scraping of the nail and look under a microscope for signs of fungus.bIn some cases, your doctor may send the sample to a lab for analysis and identification.

How is a fungal nail infection treated?

Over-the-counter products aren't usually recommended to treat nail infections since they don't provide reliable results. Instead, your doctor may prescribe an oral antifungal medication, such as:

terbinafine (Lamisil)

itraconazole (Sporanox)

fluconazole (Diflucan)

griseofulvin (Gris-PEG)

Your doctor may prescribe other antifungal treatments, such as antifungal nail lacquer or topical solutions. These treatments are brushed onto the nail in the same way that you'd apply nail polish. Depending on the type of fungus causing the infection, as well as the extent of the infection, you may have to use these medications for several months. Topical solutions aren't generally effective in curing toenail fungal infections.

Treatment isn't guaranteedTrusted Source to completely rid your body of the fungal infection. Complications from fungal infection are also possible.

Tips to prevent fungal nail infections

Making a few simple lifestyle changes can help prevent a fungal infection of the nails. Taking good care of your nails by keeping them well trimmed and clean is a good way to prevent infections.

Also avoid injuring the skin around your nails. If you're going to have damp or wet hands for an extended amount of time, you may want to wear rubber gloves. Other ways to prevent fungal infections of the nails include:

. washing your hands after touching infected nails

drying your feet well after showering, especially between your toes

getting manicures or pedicures from trustworthy salons

avoiding being barefoot in public places

reducing your use of artificial nails and nail polish

If you're prone to excessive moisture around your fingernails or toenails, consider buying:

antifungal sprays or powders

moisture-wicking socks

your own manicure or pedicure set

Long-term outlook

For some people, a fungal nail infection can be difficult to cure, and the first round of medication might not work. The nail infection can't be considered cured until a new nail that's free from infection has grown in. Although this indicates that the nail is no longer infected, it's possible for the fungal infection to return. In severe cases, there may be permanent damage to your nail, and it may have to be removed. The main complications of a fungal nail infection are:

a resurgence of the infection

a permanent loss of the affected nail

a discoloration of the infected nail

the spread of infection to other areas of the body and possibly the bloodstream

the development of a bacterial skin infection called cellulitis

It's especially important to see your doctor if you have diabetes and a fungal nail infection. People with diabetes have a greater risk for developing potentially serious complications caused by these infections. Talk to your doctor if you have diabetes and think you're developing a fungal nail infection.

What causes nail fungus to form under acrylic nails?

Fungal infections make up more than 50 percentTrusted Source of all nail disorders and are particularly common in people with acrylic nails. One studyTrusted Source found that out of a group of 68 women who developed nail concerns after removing acrylic nails, 67 of them had fungal infections. Acrylic nails are attached to your real nails with an adhesive. If they become loose or aren't put on properly, moisture can get trapped between them and your fingernails. Fungi thrive in moist environments and may start to grow around the trapped water. A group of fungi called dermatophytes are most commonly responsible for nail fungal infections, particularly the fungus Trichophyton rubrum.

Nail polish and contaminated equipment

A 2018 studyTrusted Source found evidence that fungi may be able to live and multiply in some nail polishes. It may be a good idea to avoid sharing nail polish. Contaminated equipment at a nail salon can also expose you to types of fungi that may lead to an infection.

Symptoms of fungus on fingernails from acrylic nails

Your fungal infection may not cause any symptoms in the beginning, until it progresses. As the infection gets worse, you may experience:

a brittle or thickened nail

a bad smell coming from the nail

pain and soreness, especially when putting pressure on your nail

a yellow, green, black, or white discoloration

itchiness

redness

swelling

How to get rid of a fingernail fungus from acrylic nails

Fingernail infections often clear up on their own or with home remedies. Antifungal medications are used for more serious infections.

Acrylic nail fungus home remedies

The first step after noticing an infection is to have the acrylic nail removed and to wash your fingernail with soap and water. Avoid putting on a new nail until the infection clears. Anecdotally, some people claim the following home remedies have helped them clear their infection:

Vinegar. Vinegar contains acid that can inhibit the growth of fungi and bacteria. Try soaking your finger in a 2:1 ratio of warm water to vinegar.

Vicks VapoRub. An older 2011 study found Vicks VapoRub seemed to have a positive clinical effect on killing toenail fungi. You can try applying a small amount to your finger once a day.

Tea tree oil. According to the National Center for Complementary and Integrative HealthTrusted Source, one small study found evidence that tea tree oil may help treat nail fungus, but more research is needed. Try applying oil to your nail twice per day.

Oregano oil. The chemical thymol found in oregano oil may have antifungal properties. Try applying oregano oil to your nail twice per day with a cotton swab.

Listerine mouthwash. Listerine contains ingredients that have antifungal properties. Some people claim soaking your finger in original Listerine for 30 minutes a day may help clear the infection.

Medical treatment

Medical treatment usually isn't needed for a nail fungal infection unless it becomes severe. Severe fungal infections are most common in people with suppressed immune systems, such as people undergoing chemotherapy or living with HIV. The gold standard treatment is the oral antifungal medication terbinafine. Terbinafine is only available with a prescription. You may need to use it for up to several months. A doctor may also prescribe other antifungal medications, such as:

itraconazole

fluconazole

griseofulvin

When to see a doctor

Most nail fungal infections will clear up on their own or in combination with home remedies. But it's a good idea to visit a doctor for an antifungal prescription if home remedies aren't effective or if it's causing you serious discomfort. People who are immunosuppressed may also want to visit their doctor for treatment to avoid developing a more serious infection.

Preventing acrylic nail fungus

Here are some ways you can prevent fungal infections with acrylic nails:

Get your nails put on at a reputable salon that follows good hygiene habits.

Dry your nails well after bathing or swimming.

Keep your hands dry as much as possible.

If you're prone to fungal infection, consider using an antifungal spray or powder on your nails.

Avoid putting sharp objects under your nails.

Other risks posed by acrylic nails

Other potential risks of acrylic nails include the following:

Bacterial infection

Bacterial infections aren't as common as fungal infections, but people with artificial fingernails tend to be more prone to developing bacterial nail infections than people without fake nails. Staphylococcus aureus and streptococci bacteria are two of the most common causes of bacterial nail infections.

Allergic reaction

It's possible to have an allergic reaction to acylates or the adhesive used to bind your nails. Allergic reactions are usually contained to the area around the nail and may cause symptoms like:

dry or flaky skin around the nail

redness

itchiness

swelling

Weakened nails

For acrylic nails to stick, your real nails need to be filed down. This filing thins your nail and can make it more brittle. Acetone is often used to remove acrylic nails, which can contribute to nail brittleness or dryness.

Takeaway

Fungal infections are a common complication of acrylic nails. They are usually caused by moisture trapped under your nails that leads to excessive fungi growth. Most fungal infections aren't serious and can be treated at home. More serious infections usually clear up with prescription antifungal medications.

Why You Shouldn't Use Bleach to Get Rid of Toenail Fungus

Toenail fungus can turn an otherwise healthy toenail into a discolored, thickened, and cracking one. While fungal toenail infections may be fairly common, this doesn't mean you should use common household products — like bleach — to treat the infection. Keep reading to find out why bleach is a bad idea for your toenail fungus, and what doctors recommend you use instead to treat it.

Dangers of using bleach for toenail fungus

Bleach (sodium hypochlorite) may actually cause toenail fungus to worsen and increase the likelihood of a toenail infection. According to an article in the Asian Journal of Research in Dermatological Science, use of topical bleach can increase the risks for fungal infections because it can damage the skin and nails. This allows opportunistic fungus to come in through the damaged skin or nail and cause an infection.

Topical bleach warnings

Never apply concentrated (undiluted) bleach to the skin. It can create a painful chemical burn that may require medical attention. Breathing in concentrated bleach fumes can also damage your lungs. If you do get bleach accidentally on your skin, quickly rinse the bleach away with water.

What about bleach baths?

Bleach baths are an approach dermatologists may recommend for treating skin conditions such as atopic dermatitis and recurrent Staphylococcus infections on the skin. These involve mixing a very small amount of bleach in bath water — typically a half cup of bleach to a full-sized bathtub of water. While it's true that bleach baths may temporarily kill bacteria, fungi, and viruses, the effects aren't long-lasting and aren't likely to treat an existing toenail fungal infection.

Bleach bath precautions

You shouldn't take a bleach bath unless a doctor recommends it. This is because bleach baths can irritate and dry out the skin for people who don't really need the approach. Also, the bleach can worsen conditions like asthma. Accidentally drinking bleach can burn the mouth and throat as well as lead to severe stomach upset and bleeding.

Potential safe uses for bleach

The myth that bleach could treat toenail fungus may be less related to topical applications and more about using bleach to clean other items that could potentially infect the toenails, such as nail clippers or files. Shoes and socks exposed to toenail fungus can be washed with bleach. Follow the bleach product's directions for your washer and laundry load size. You can also use bleach-based solutions to clean areas where fungus may grow in your home, such as your shower tiles, bath mats, or floor.

Wear gloves when handling bleach

Always wear gloves when handling bleach and mix any bleach solutions in a well-ventilated area. Don't mix bleach with other household cleansers — only water.

How to safely treat toenail fungus

Now that you know bleach isn't an effective toenail fungus treatment, let's look at some options that are.

Antifungal medications

Most of the time, you'll need to see a doctor for a prescription antifungal medication, such as terbinafine or itraconazole. These will often involve taking a pill that helps to kill the fungus. Sometimes, you may have to take these pills over an extended time period (12 weeks or more) before you see improvements in your toenail. However, oral antifungal medications can have potentially severe side effects. A doctor should review these effects with you to determine if this treatment approach is right for you and your overall health.

Laser therapy

If you don't want to take antifungal medications, or your doctor is concerned with how well they may work, laser therapy is another option. Laser treatments involve applying a photosensitizing compound to the toenail and exposing the toenail to laser light. This has the effect of killing off fungus or keeping it from multiplying.

Toenail removal/debridement

When a doctor is treating your infected toenail, they may debride the nail or remove the outer most, damaged layers. Only a professional should do this to prevent further damage to your nail. In rare instances when the toenail fungus has severely damaged your toenail, a doctor may recommend removing the nail.

Unfortunately, the warm and moist environment inside your shoe can make you vulnerable to fungal infections. When these occur on the toenail, doctors call the condition onychomycosis. Fungal skin infections commonly called athlete's foot can often affect the foot as well. One of the most common waysTrusted Source you get a fungal toenail infection is when fungus invades small cracks in your toenail. Some people are at greater risk for this occurring, including those with:

circulation problems, especially related to the feet

diabetes

history of injury, surgery, or damage to the nail

impacted immune system function

Preventative steps to take

While you can't always help your risk factors for toenail fungus, there are some preventive steps you can take:

Bring your own sterilized instruments, such as nail clippers, to a nail salon.

Keep your toenails short and clean to prevent nail trauma that can lead to cracking. If you have difficulty trimming your own toenails, your doctor may recommend seeing a podiatrist to help.

Don't share personal care items like fingernail clippers or pumice stones with another person.

Throw away or treat potentially infected footwear.

Wear clean socks and wash socks after use.

Wear sandals when walking in a locker room, public shower, or any other places where fungus is likely to grow.

Toenail fungal infections have a high rate of recurrence, even after you've treated them. That's why it's important to couple treatment measures with preventive ones to give yourself the best chance for keeping your toenails healthy in appearance.

Takeaway

Bleach isn't a good method for treating or preventing toenail fungus. Bleach can burn the skin and shouldn't be applied (even in highly diluted amounts) unless a doctor recommends it. Fungus infections often require oral medications or specialized laser treatments. Even then, the infection can come back. If you're concerned about a fungal nail infection, talk to a doctor about the most effective treatments for you.

IS TEA TREE OIL A SAFE AND EFFECTIVE TREATMENT FOR NAIL FUNGUS?

Tea tree oil may help to clear up nail fungus when applied regularly, but it may be a while before you notice an improvement. Tea tree oil is an essential oil with many therapeutic benefits. Among its healing benefits, tea tree oil has antifungal and antiseptic propertiesTrusted Source and may be an effective treatment for nail fungus. Nail fungus can be challenging to treat because it may not resolve right away. If you use tea tree oil consistently, you should see results over time. Just keep in mind that the results won't be immediate.

Does tea tree oil work?

Results from scientific studies supporting the use of tea tree oil to treat nail fungus are mixed. Some of the research points to tea tree oil's potential as an antifungal, but more studies are needed. According to a 2013 study, tea tree oil was effective in reducing growth of the fungus Trichophyton rubrum in nail infections. T. rubrum is a fungus that can cause infections such as athlete's foot and nail fungus. Improvements were seen after 14 days. This study used an in vitro model, which is sometimes called a test-tube experiment. In in vitro studies, the experiment is done in a test tube instead of on an animal or human. Larger human studies are needed to expand on these findings.

Combining tea tree oil with standard medicated creams is also an option. A small 1999 studyTrusted Source found that participants were able to successfully manage toenail fungus by using a cream that contained butenafine hydrochloride and tea tree oil. After 16 weeks of treatment, 80 percent of participants who used this cream cured their toenail fungus with no relapses. No one in the placebo group cured their nail fungus. Further studies are needed to determine which of these ingredients is most useful in treating nail fungus. Results of a 1994 studyTrusted Source found pure tea tree oil was equally as effective as the antifungal clotrimazole (Desenex) in treating fungal toenail infections. Clotrimazole is available both over the counter (OTC) and by prescription.

After six months of twice-daily treatment, results of both groups were similar. While both groups had positive results, recurrence was common. Further studies are needed to determine how to treat nail fungus with no recurrence.

Is it safe?

It's generally safe to use tea tree oil topically, but no more than 3 drops directly to the skin. If you have sensitive skin you may experience dryness, itching, stinging, redness or burning. It's always best to do a skin test prior to use by testing with one drop of tea tree oil.

For every 1 to 2 drops of tea tree oil, add 12 drops of a carrier oil.

Apply a dime-sized amount of the diluted oil to your forearm.

If you don't experience any irritation within 24 hours, it should be safe to apply elsewhere.

Never take tea tree oil internally. Avoid using tea tree oil on children without consulting a doctor. Tea tree essential oils can be diluted in a carrier oil, such as sweet almond oil or coconut oil. It's possible for tea tree oil to cause an allergic reaction. It can cause skin irritation such as redness, itchiness, and inflammation in some people. Talk to your doctor before using tea tree oil if you're pregnant or breastfeeding.

How to use

Tea tree oil is easy to use. If you are using the tea tree oil undiluted, or "neat", do a patch test first. Then use up to 3 drops of undiluted tea tree essential oil directly on the fungus. If you are diluting the tea tree oil, add it to a carrier oil, such as coconut oil. You can either use a cotton swab to apply it and allow it to dry or place a cotton ball soaked in the diluted tea tree oil on the affected area for a few minutes. You can also do a foot soak a few times per week. Add five drops of tea tree oil to a half-ounce of carrier oil, mix them, stir into a bucket of warm water, and soak your feet for 20 minutes.

Keep your nails neat and nicely trimmed during the healing process. Use clean nail clippers, scissors, or a nail file to remove any dead nails. Also, keep your affected nails as clean and dry as possible. Always wash your hands thoroughly after treating your nails to avoid spreading the infection.

How long does it take to recover?

You need to be consistent with the treatment in order to see results. It usually takes a few months for the nail to heal completely. Healing time depends on how severe the infection is and how quickly your body responds to the treatment. The fungal infection is cured when you've grown an entirely new nail that's free from infection. You can continue the tea tree oil treatment after the nail has healed to ensure that the nail fungus doesn't return.

Buying essential oils

It's important that you use a high-quality tea tree oil for best results. Here are some things to look for when buying tea tree oil:

The oil needs to be 100 percent pure.

Buy an organic oil, if possible.

Look for a tea tree oil that has a 10 to 40 percent concentration of terpinen. This is one of the main antiseptic and antifungal components of tea tree oil.

You can buy tea tree oil online or at a local health store. Always buy from a brand that you trust. The supplier should be able to answer any questions you have about their product. Research your brands and manufacturers. Essential oils can have issues with purity, contamination, and strength. The U. S. Food and Drug Administration (FDA) doesn't regulate essential oils, so it's important to purchase from a supplier you trust.

How to store essential oils

Store your essential oils away from direct sunlight, moisture, and extreme temperatures. They should be okay at room temperature. If you live in a very warm or humid climate, you can store them in the refrigerator.

When to seek help

If you've taken steps to treat your nail fungus but it isn't improving or starts to get worse, it's important that you see a doctor. Nail fungus has the potential to cause other complications, especially for people who have diabetes or a weakened immune system.

Using tea tree oil should be a safe and effective method for treating nail fungus, but it's still important that you use it with care. Keep an eye on the effect it's having on your nail fungus and possibly on the skin around it. Discontinue use immediately if you experience any adverse effects. Also keep in mind that it may take some time to completely heal nail fungus.

Recognizing the Symptoms of Yellow Nail Syndrome

Yellow nail syndrome is a rare condition that affects the fingernails and toenails. People who develop this condition also have respiratory problems and lymphatic system problems with swelling in the lower parts of their body. Swelling is caused by a buildup of lymph under the soft tissue of the skin. Lymph is a colorless fluid that circulates throughout your body and helps cleanse it. Yellow nail syndrome can occur in anyone, but usually occurs in adults over the age of 50.

What are symptoms of yellow nail syndrome?

Yellow nail syndrome is when nails gradually turn yellow and thicken. Symptoms also include:

the loss of the cuticle, which is part of the protective skin covering the nail

nails that curve

nails that stop growing

nails that separate from the nail bed

nail loss

Yellow nail syndrome sometimes increases the risk for an infection around the soft tissue of the nails. Fluid accumulation often accompanies yellow nail syndrome. So you may develop fluid between the membranes that surround the outside of your lungs, a condition known as pleural effusion. This can cause several respiratory problems, such as:

chronic cough

shortness of breath

chest pains

Respiratory problems may occur before or after your nails begin to change in color and shape. In addition to having a pleural effusion and its associated respiratory difficulty, other breathing problems may occur in yellow nail syndrome. These include chronic sinusitis or recurrent respiratory infections such as pneumonia.

Lymphedema is also associated with yellow nail syndrome. This condition arises from an accumulation of lymph. Signs include swelling mainly in your legs, but possibly also in your arms.

What are the causes of yellow nail syndrome?

The exact cause of yellow nail syndrome is unknown.. This condition can start sporadically for no apparent reason, which occurs in most cases. Even so, in rare cases, it's believed it may run in families. A mutation of the FOXC2 gene — which causes a disorder called lymphedema-distichiasis syndrome — may play a role in developing yellow nail syndrome. More research is needed to confirm this, as other literature currently reports that there is no known genetic factor for yellow nail syndrome.

Another belief is that yellow nail syndrome results from problems with lymphatic drainage. Improper circulation and drainage of lymph allows fluid to collect in the soft tissue under the skin, which may slowly turn nails yellow. Yellow nail syndrome can also develop on its own or occur with certain types of cancers, autoimmune diseases like rheumatoid arthritis, and immunodeficiencies.

How to diagnose yellow nail syndrome?

You shouldn't ignore a change in nail color or shape, especially if your nails turn yellow. Yellow nails can indicate a problem with your liver or kidney, diabetes mellitus, fungal infections, or psoriasis, which need to be treated by a doctor. If you develop yellow nails along with swelling or respiratory problems, see a doctor. A doctor may diagnose yellow nail syndrome if you exhibit primary symptoms of the condition. Your doctor may also order a pulmonary function test to measure how well your lungs work or take a sample of your nail to check for fungus.

Complications of yellow nail syndrome

Yellow nail syndrome is also associated with bronchiectasis, which is when the small airways in your lung become abnormally widened, weak, and scarred. In bronchiectasis, airway mucus can't be properly moved. As a result, you could end up developing pneumonia if your lungs fill up with germy mucus and become infected. This bronchiectasis, in addition to the fluid that builds up in the pleural space outside of the lungs, causes lung problems.

Treatment for yellow nail syndrome

There's no one treatment for yellow nail syndrome. Treatment addresses specific symptoms of the condition and may include:

topical or oral vitamin E for nail discoloration

corticosteroids

oral zinc

antifungal medications

antibiotics in the case of bacterial sinusitis, lung infections, or excess mucus production

diuretics, which remove excess fluid

tube thoracostomy, a procedure to drain fluid from the pleural space

If yellow nail syndrome occurs with an associated disease like cancer, arthritis, or AIDS, symptoms may improve after treating the underlying disease. To treat lymphedema-distichiasis syndrome, your doctor may recommend manual lymph drainage, which is a specialized massage technique to improve circulation and reduce puffiness. You can also reduce lymphedema at home by wearing elastic compression garments. Compression encourages better lymph flow through your lymphatic vessels.

Outlook and prevention

There's no way to prevent yellow nail syndrome, but the symptoms can be manageable with medication, fluid removal, and supplementation. As lymph drainage improves, nails may return to a normal color. One study found that nail symptom improvement may occur in 7 to 30 percent of those with yellow nail syndrome. Because lymphedema can become a chronic condition, some people require ongoing therapy to manage swelling and fluid accumulation.

TRY ONE OF THESE 10 HOME REMEDIES FOR TOENAIL FUNGUS

You may be able to treat toenail fungus at home with certain essential oils and other products with antimicrobial and antifungal properties. fungus, also called onychomycosis, is a common fungal infection of the toenail. The most noticeable symptom is a white, brown, or yellow discoloration of one or more of the toenails. It may spread and cause the nails to thicken or crack. Sandal season or not, toenail fungus typically isn't what you want to see when you look at your feet. There are many treatments you can try, and some of them can be natural. Here are 10 at-home treatments for toenail fungus:

1. Vicks VapoRub

Vicks VapoRub is a topical ointment. Although designed for cough suppression, its active ingredients (camphor and eucalyptus oil) may help treat toenail fungus. An older 2011 study found that Vicks VapoRub had a "positive clinical effect" in treating toenail fungus. Another 2016 studyTrusted Source on living with HIV confirmed this finding. To use, apply a small amount of Vicks VapoRub to the affected area at least once a day.

2. Snakeroot extract

Snakeroot (Ageratina pichinchensis) extract is an antifungal made from plants in the sunflower family. An older 2008 study showed that the remedy is effective against toenail fungus as the antifungal medication ciclopirox. For the study, snakeroot extract was applied to the affected area every third day for the first month, twice a week for the second month, and once a week for the third month. A 2020 studyTrusted Source on people living with diabetes mellitus confirmed these findings.

3. Tea tree oil

Tea tree oil, also called melaleuca, is an essential oil with antifungal and antiseptic abilities. According to the

National Center for Complementary and Integrative HealthTrusted Source (NCCIH), some small-scale clinical studies showed that tea tree oil might be effective against toenail fungus. Paint the tea tree oil directly onto the affected nail twice daily with a cotton swab.

4. Oregano oil

Oregano oil contains thymol. According to a 2016 review, thymol has antifungal and antibacterial properties. To treat toenail fungus, apply oregano oil to the affected nail twice daily with a cotton swab. Some people use oregano oil and tea tree oil together. Both products are potent and may cause irritation or allergic reactions. Combining them may increase this risk.

5. Ozonized oils

Ozonized oils are oils like olive oil and sunflower oil that are "injected" with ozone gas. According to research from 2020Trusted Source, this type of ozone exposure in low concentrations for a short duration can then inactivate many organisms, such as fungi, yeast, and bacteria.

6. Listerine mouthwash

Listerine mouthwash can help treat toenail fungus because it contains menthol, thymol, and eucalyptus, which have antibacterial and antifungal properties. This may be why it's a popular folk remedy for toenail fungus. Supporters of the treatment recommend soaking the affected foot in a basin of amber-colored Listerine for 30 minutes daily.

7. Garlic

A study from 2019Trusted Source suggests that garlic extract could have antifungal properties, but more research is needed to confirm this. You may treat toenail fungus with garlic by placing chopped or crushed garlic cloves on the affected area for 30 minutes daily. It may be better, and less smelly, to treat it from the inside out with garlic capsules. Take as directed by the manufacturer.

8. Apple cider vinegar

Only anecdotal evidence exists supporting vinegar as a treatment for toenail fungus. There is one 2017 study on apple cider vinegar suggesting it has antimicrobial properties. That said, more research is needed on its actual effect on toenail fungus. If you want to give vinegar a try, soak the affected foot in one part vinegar to two parts warm water for up to 20 minutes daily.

9. Probiotics

ResearchTrusted Source shows that probiotics may help prevent the growth of various fungi, which may be able to reduce the chance of an infection. Consider eating more foods containing probiotics or taking probiotic supplements as a preventive strategy.

10. Other natural options

The are a few other plant-based remedies that may be effective in treating toenail fungus, according to research. These include:

spirulina (Arthrospira maxima)

spruce tree resin

propolis extract

When to see a doctor

In most cases, toenail fungus is considered a cosmetic problem. Still, it may cause serious complications for some people. People living with diabetes have a greater chanceTrusted Source of getting toenail fungus. Infections may, in turn, contribute to the development of a diabetic foot ulcer. You shouldn't use home remedies for toenail fungus if you have diabetes or a weakened immune system. Contact your doctor for the appropriate course of action.

How do you get rid of toenail fungus fast at home?

If you want to get rid of a toenail fungus quickly, the best thing to do is to see a doctor for prescription medication such as fluconazole (Diflucan). Natural remedies may be able to relieve your symptoms, but there isn't certainty that they will work, and even if they do, it will likely take longer.

What absolutely kills toenail fungus?

Prescription oral antifungals, such as terbinafine (Lamisil) or fluconazole (Diflucan), are traditionally used to treat toenail fungus and will usually resolve it faster and more effectively. On the other hand, they can also cause serious side effects such as upset stomach, dizziness, severe skin problems, and jaundice. This may be why many people try home remedies instead.

Does hydrogen peroxide help toenail fungus?

According to a study, a new medication A3IS (Mycosinate)Trusted Source that slowly releases hydrogen peroxide was found to be about 40% more effective than Amorolfine (Curanail, Loceryl, Locetar, and Odenil) after 6-12 weeks of treatment, and 70% more effective at 6 months of treatment. That said, Mycosinate may not yet be available for commercial use. However, this research did not examine the direct application of hydrogen peroxide on toenail fungus. The Global Nail Fungus Organization does list the substance as a remedy.

Home remedies may be more effective than prescription medications in treating mild-to-moderate toenail fungus. Although home remedies typically have fewer side effects, there's less scientific evidence that they work. Many factors come into play when treating toenail fungus, such as nail penetrability, infection severity, and overall health. Home remedies may take longer to wipe out toenail fungus than topical prescription medications or oral systemic antifungals. You may not see results for several months. Reinfection is common.

Once the infection is gone, keep your toenails dry, clean, and well-trimmed. Severe cases of toenail fungus may cause pain and irreversible toenail damage. If you try home remedies to treat the infection that doesn't work or causes side effects, consult your doctor.

Tips to prevent fungal nail infections

Making a few simple lifestyle changes can help prevent a fungal infection of the nails. Taking good care of your nails by keeping them well trimmed and clean is a good way to prevent infections.nAlso avoid injuring the skin around your nails. If you're going to have damp or wet hands for an extended amount of time, you may want to wear rubber gloves.nOther ways to prevent fungal infections of the nails include:

washing your hands after touching infected nails

drying your feet well after showering, especially between your toes

getting manicures or pedicures from trustworthy salons

avoiding being barefoot in public places

reducing your use of artificial nails and nail polish

PRODUCTS TO HELP YOU AVOID NAIL FUNGUS

If you're prone to excessive moisture around your fingernails or toenails, consider buying:

antifungal sprays or powders

moisture-wicking socks

your own manicure or pedicure set

Long-term outlook

For some people, a fungal nail infection can be difficult to cure, and the first round of medication might not work. The nail infection can't be considered cured until a new nail that's free from infection has grown in.

Although this indicates that the nail is no longer infected, it's possible for the fungal infection to return. In severe cases, there may be permanent damage to your nail, and it may have to be removed.

The main complications of a fungal nail infection are:

a resurgence of the infection

a permanent loss of the affected nail

a discoloration of the infected nail

the spread of infection to other areas of the body and possibly the bloodstream

the development of a bacterial skin infection called cellulitis

It's especially important to see your doctor if you have diabetes and a fungal nail infection. People with diabetes have a greater risk for developing potentially serious complications caused by these infections. Talk to your doctor if you have diabetes and think you're developing a fungal nail infection.

CONCLUSION

In fungal infections, invasive fungi grow in or on your body. Many types of fungi occur naturally in your body in small amounts. Some infections occur when these fungi grow out of control while other infections are caused by types of fungi not normally present in your body. Fungal infections are a relatively common complication of getting acrylic nails, which are plastic nails that are glued atop your real fingernails. In most cases, these infections aren't serious and clear up with home remedies or with antifungal medications. Let's look at why acrylic nails sometimes cause fingernail fungal infections, how you can treat these infections, and how to prevent them.